We dedicate this book to all of the brave children and loved ones who have had a kidney transplant as well as the donors who make it all possible!

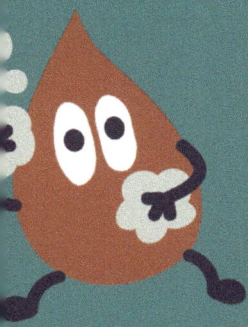
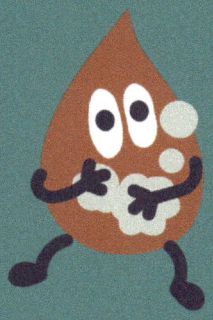
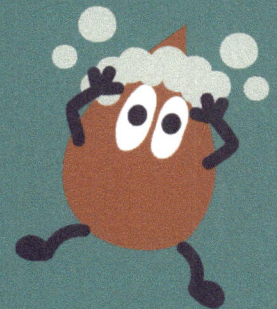
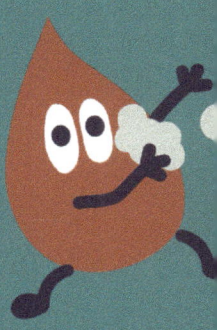

Text copyright © 2025 Child Core Family Support LLC.

All rights reserved.

No part of this book may be reproduced or transmitted in any form or by any means, electronic or mechanical, including photocopying, recording, or by any information storage and retrieval system, without written permission from the publisher.

The only exception is brief quotations for reviews.

For information please contact author at hello@childcorefamilysupport.com

ISBN: 979-8-9987553-0-9

The information in this book is based on our own education, research, and experience. It is designed to be used as a tool to support a child's understanding of the topic of a kidney transplant and not in lieu of already existing supports, consults, or medical information provided by Child Life Specialists or other medical professionals.

For more information about Child Life Specialists and how they can help your child, go to childcorefamilysupport.com.

Written + Illustrated by Adrienne O'Connor, MS, CCLS
Written by Caitlin McNamara, MS, CCLS, CIMI

Pssst... Check out pages 46 to 49 of the book for fun activities to go along with the story.

Oh hey, I didn't see you there. I was just busy checking out my kidney!

Did you know our kidneys are about the size of our fists? Go on, make a fist and see!

Let's go learn more about our kidneys.

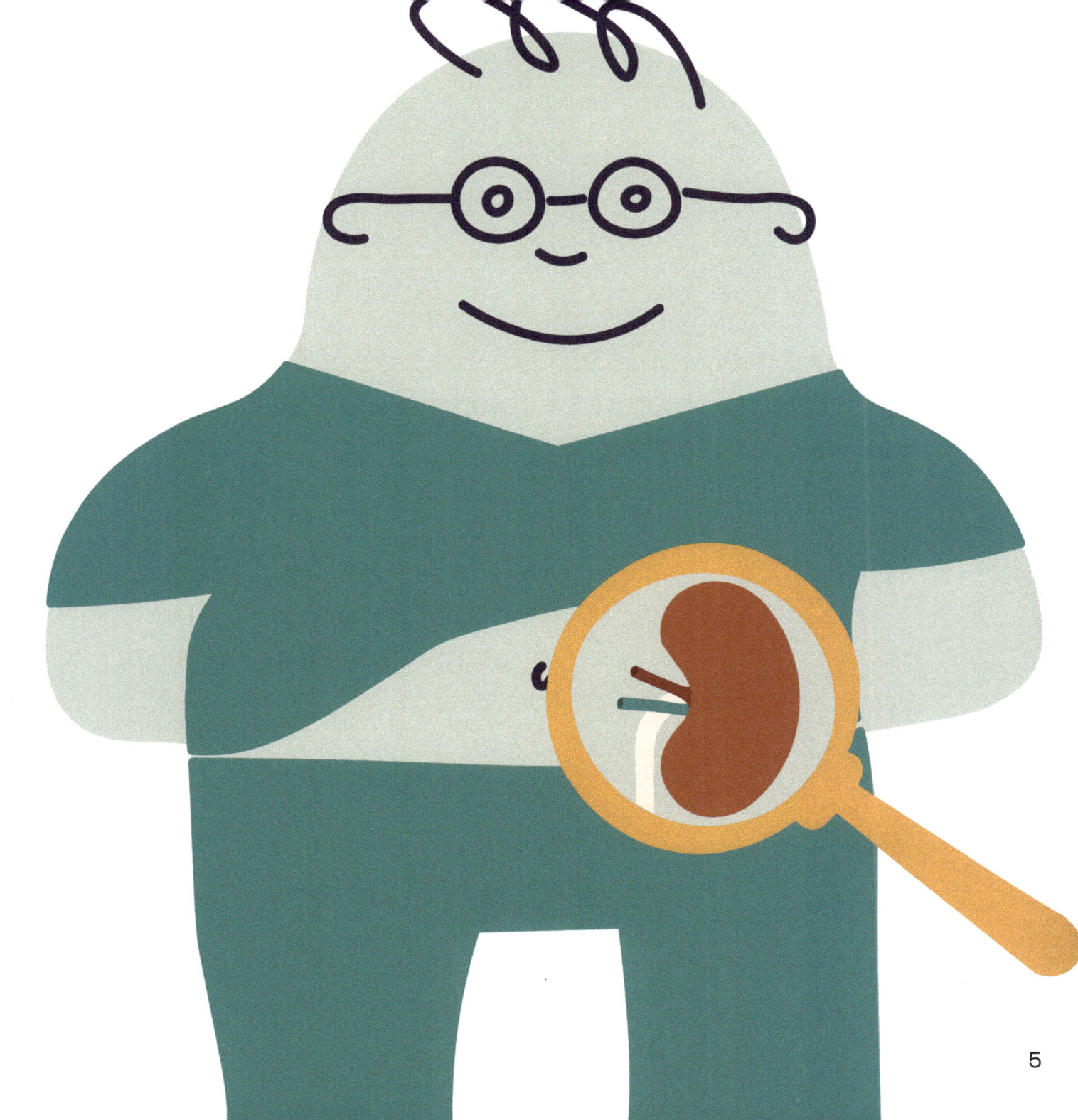

It can be helpful when learning about our kidneys, to start by taking a look at how our bodies work.

Our bodies are made up of different parts that all work together.

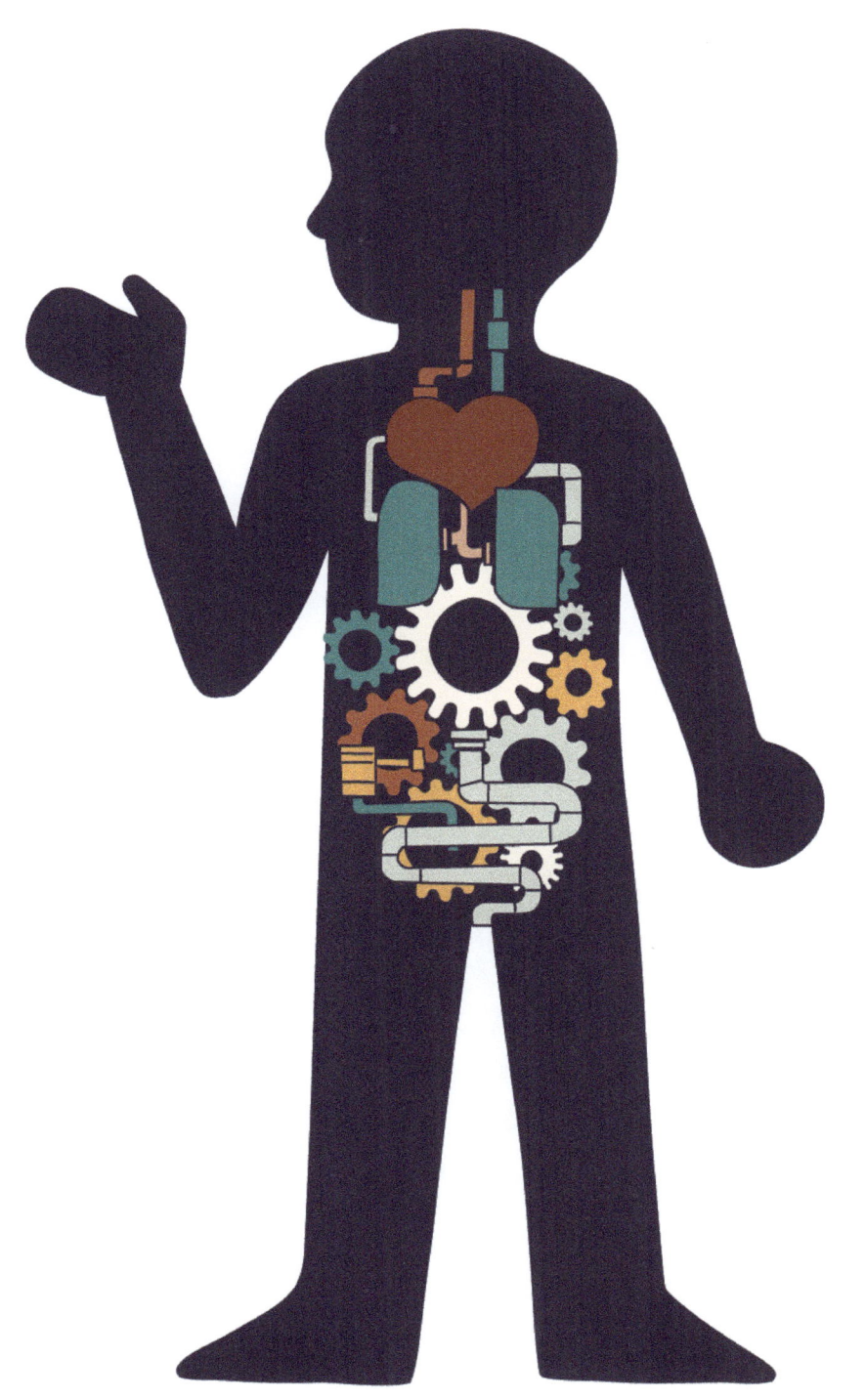

All of these parts have jobs that help our bodies do different things.

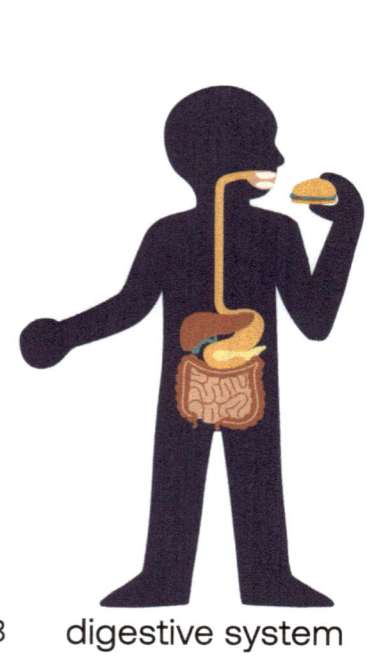
digestive system

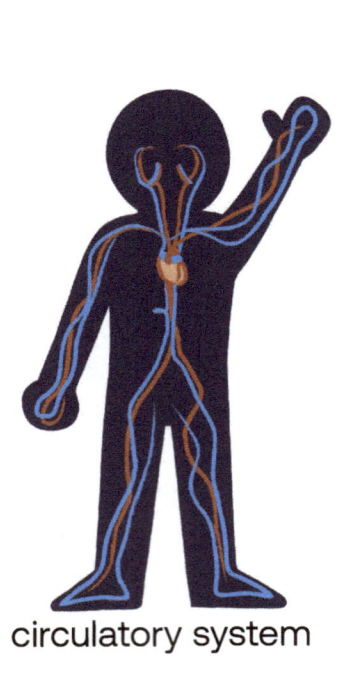
circulatory system

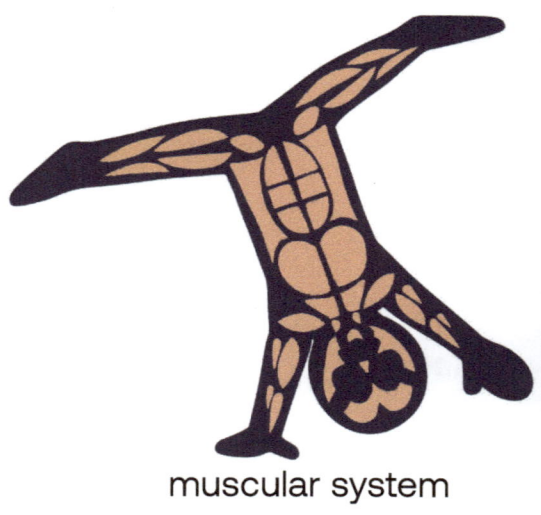
muscular system

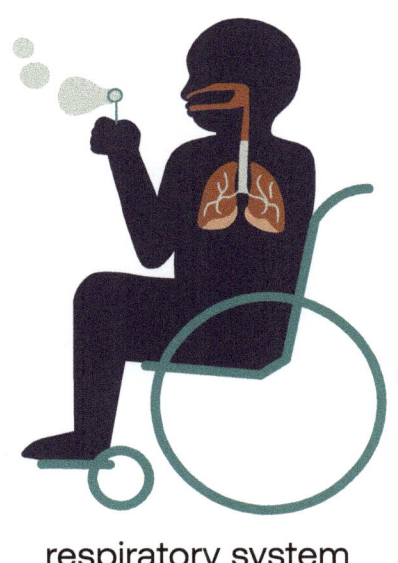
respiratory system

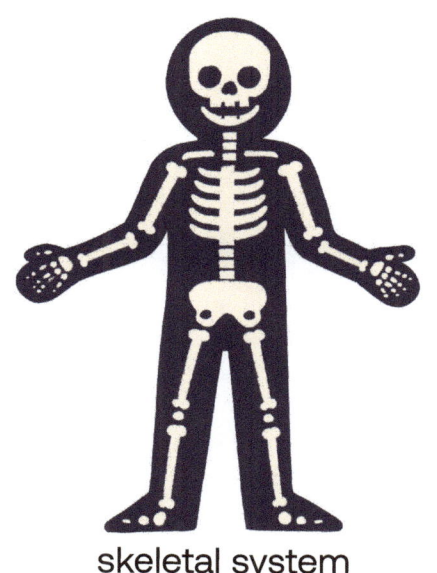
skeletal system

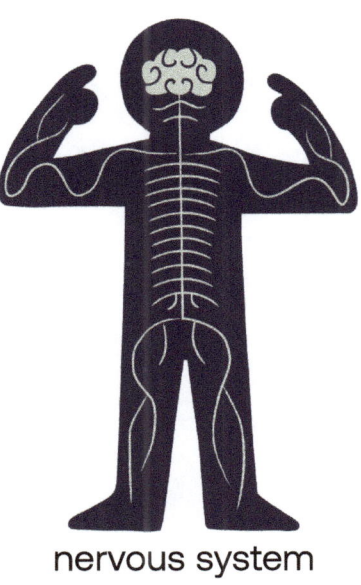
nervous system

Like being able to play, digest our food, breathe, use our imagination, and even go to the bathroom.

Now, let's introduce our kidneys.

Our kidneys work together with other body parts to
clean our blood
and
make urine (or pee).

Fun Fact: It is common for a body to have two kidneys, but sometimes a body may only need one kidney to do the job of two!

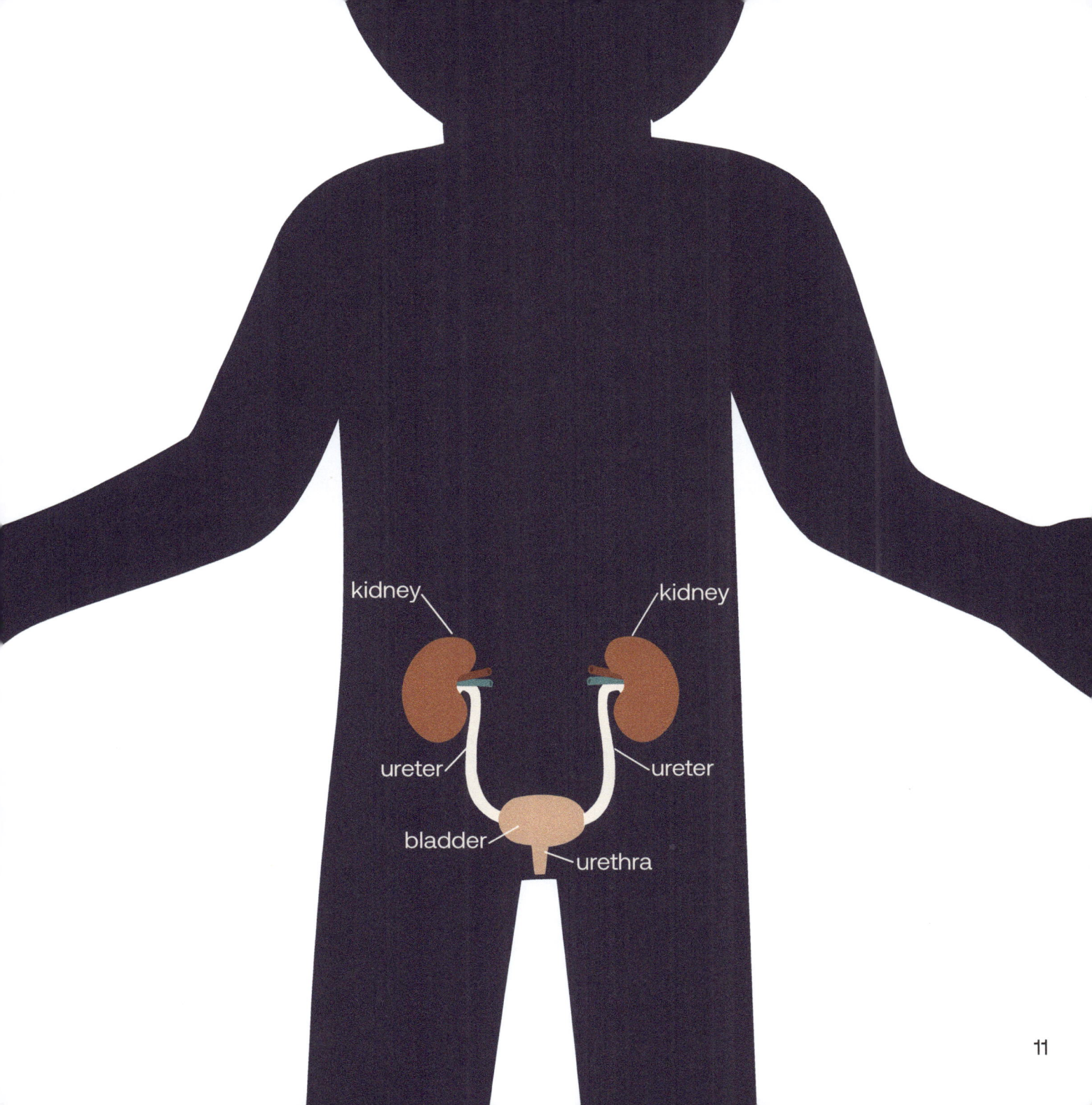

Here is a look at how this works.

As our blood travels through our body it picks up extra fluid and waste.

Then, our blood travels into our kidneys where it is cleaned by removing the extra fluid and waste.

The clean blood then exits our kidneys and travels back throughout our body. Finally, the fluid and waste leaves our body through our pee.

*see the glossary to learn more about fluid and waste.

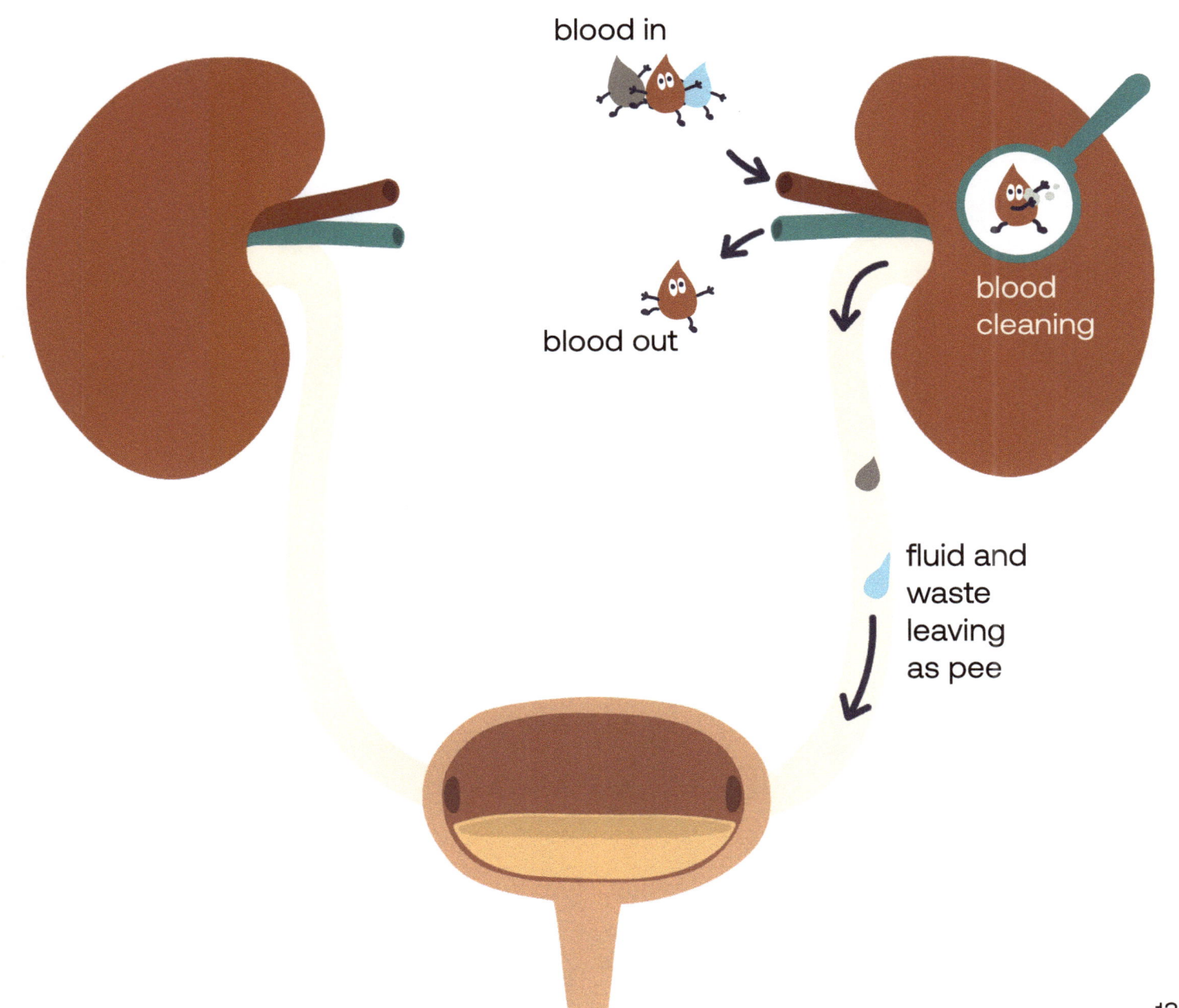

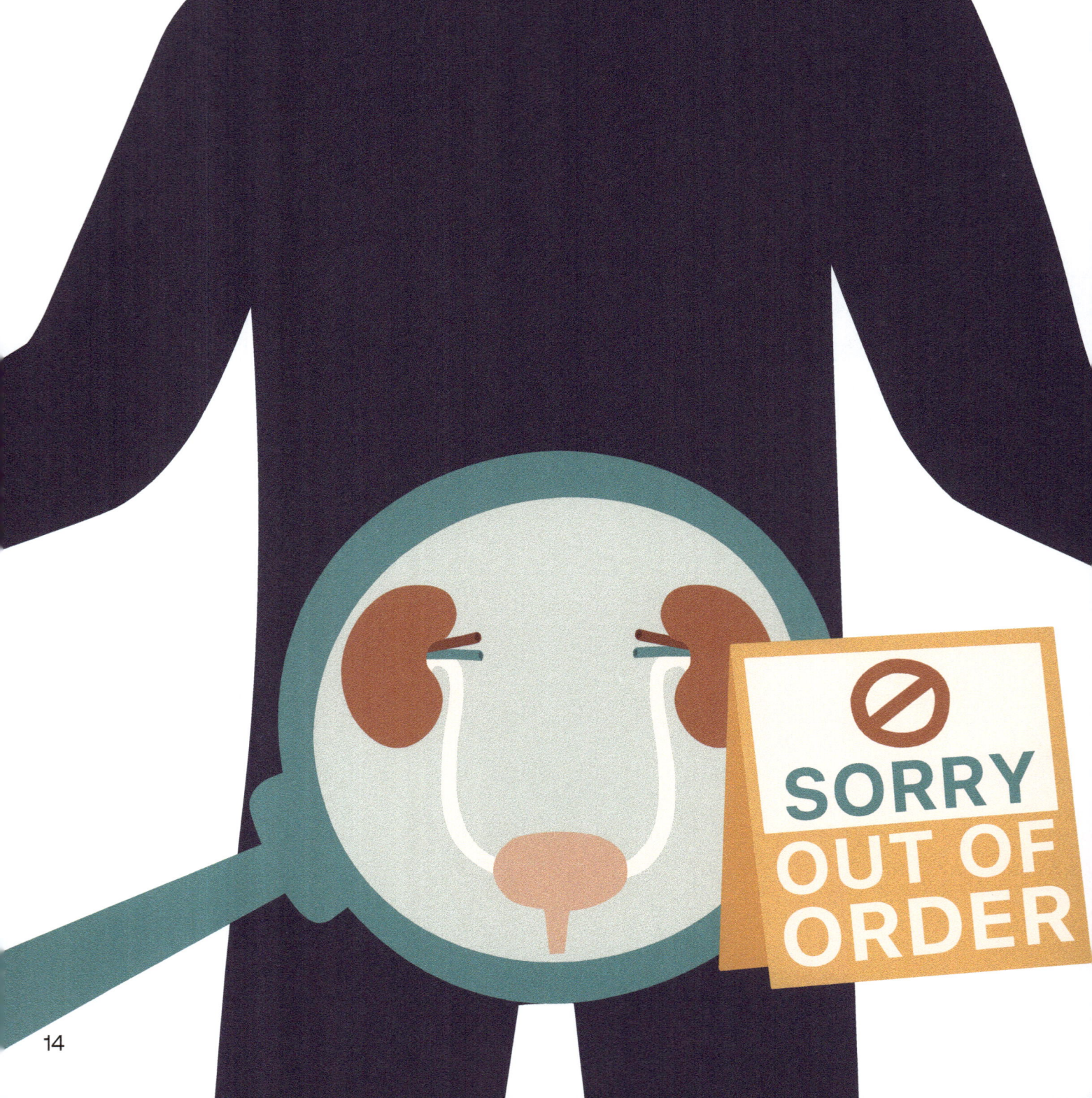

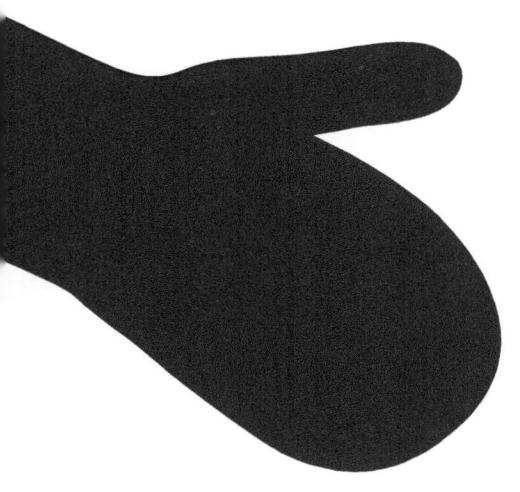

What do you think would happen if someone's kidneys can't do their job?

If someone's kidneys aren't working, their body isn't able to clean their blood and remove the extra fluid and waste.

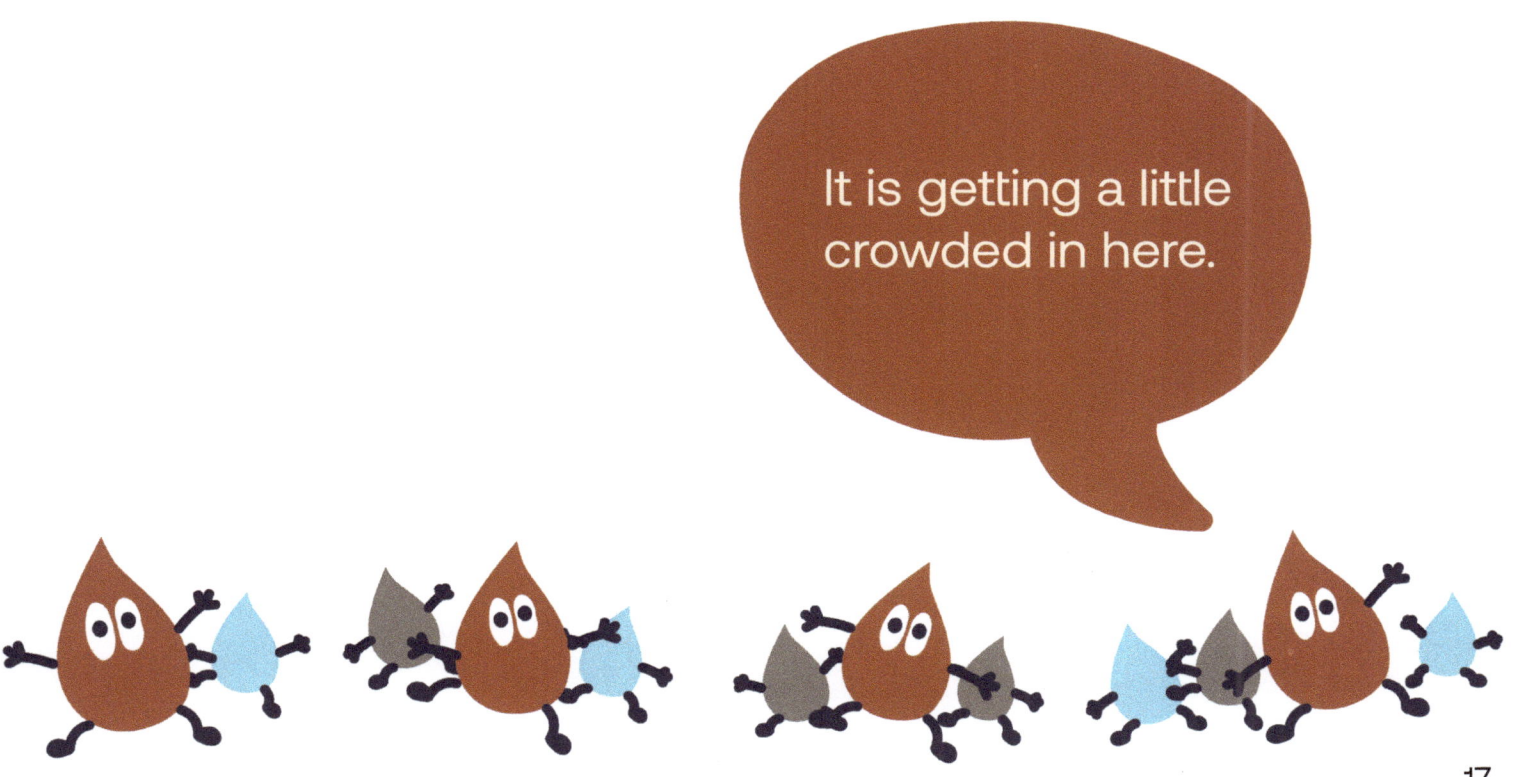

When extra fluid and waste stays in the blood, it might cause a person to...

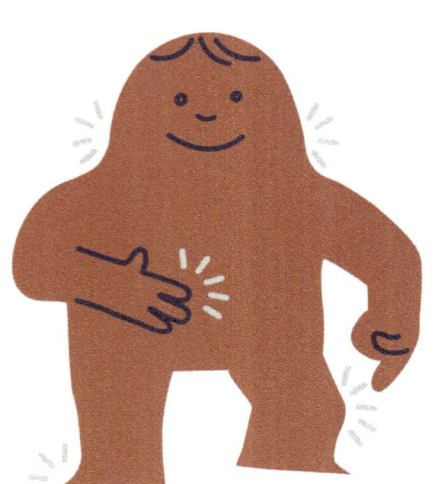

have swelling in legs, feet, hands, or face

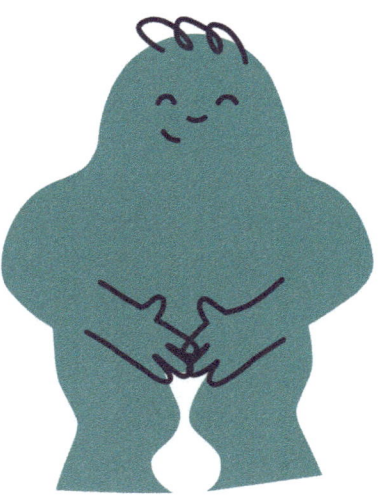

have to pee less or more

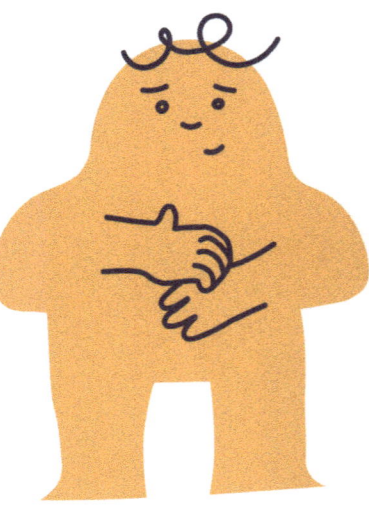

have itchy skin

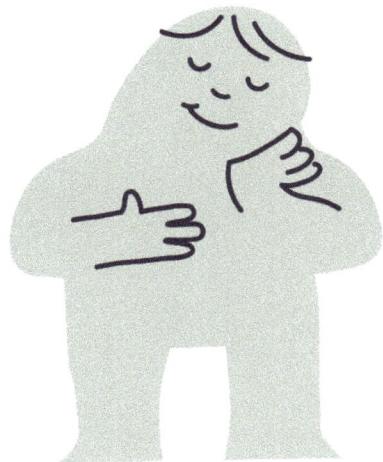

feel more tired
or weak

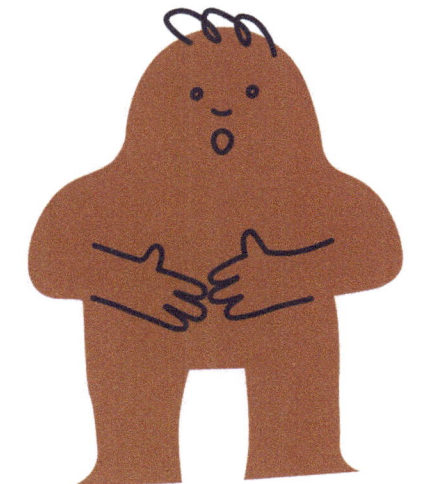

have a stomach ache

So what happens next?

When someone's kidneys aren't working, they might need to get a new kidney.

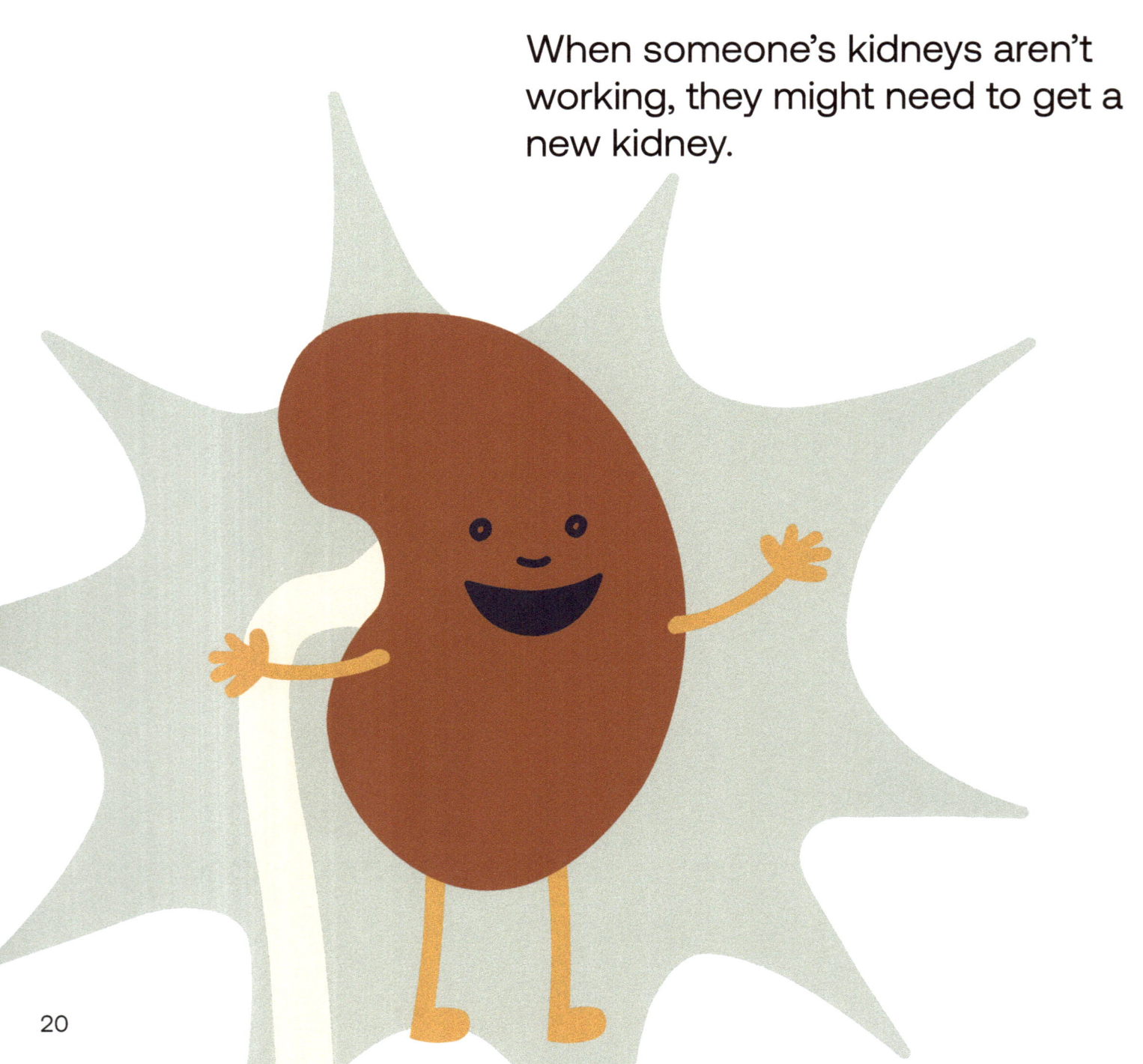

This is known as a

kidney transplant!

Transplant means getting something new. So a kidney transplant means getting a new kidney!

Can you buy a new kidney?

Nope.

Can you grow a new kidney?

Sorry, not possible.

So where does the new kidney come from?

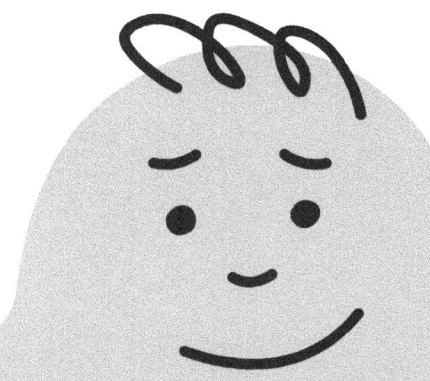

A kidney comes from another person who chooses to donate, or give, one of their kidneys!

This person is called a **donor.**

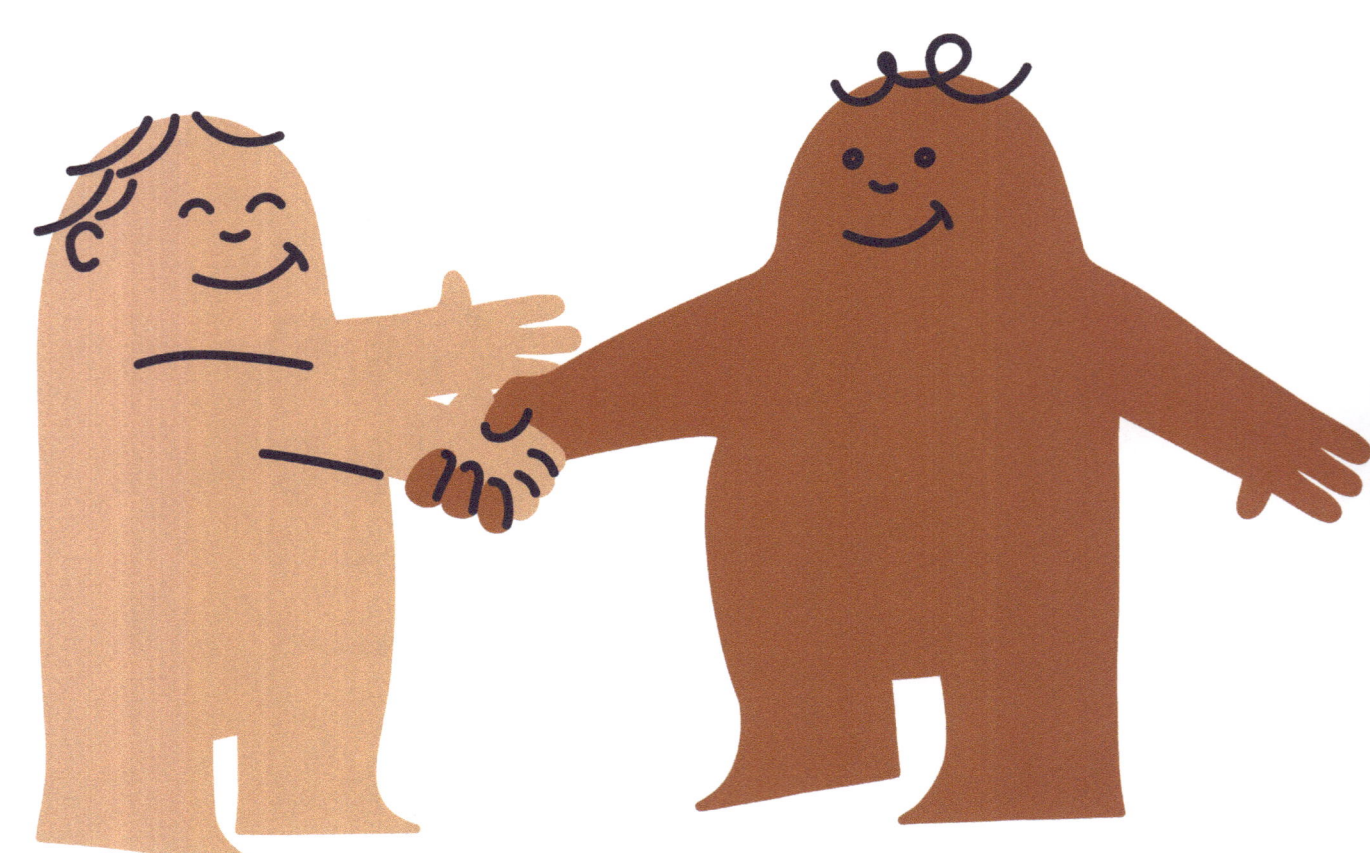

And remember, someone only needs one healthy kidney to do the job of cleaning their blood.

So, when a donor gives one of their kidneys to someone else, their remaining kidney will do the job of two.

A donor can be someone the person knows, like a family member or friend.

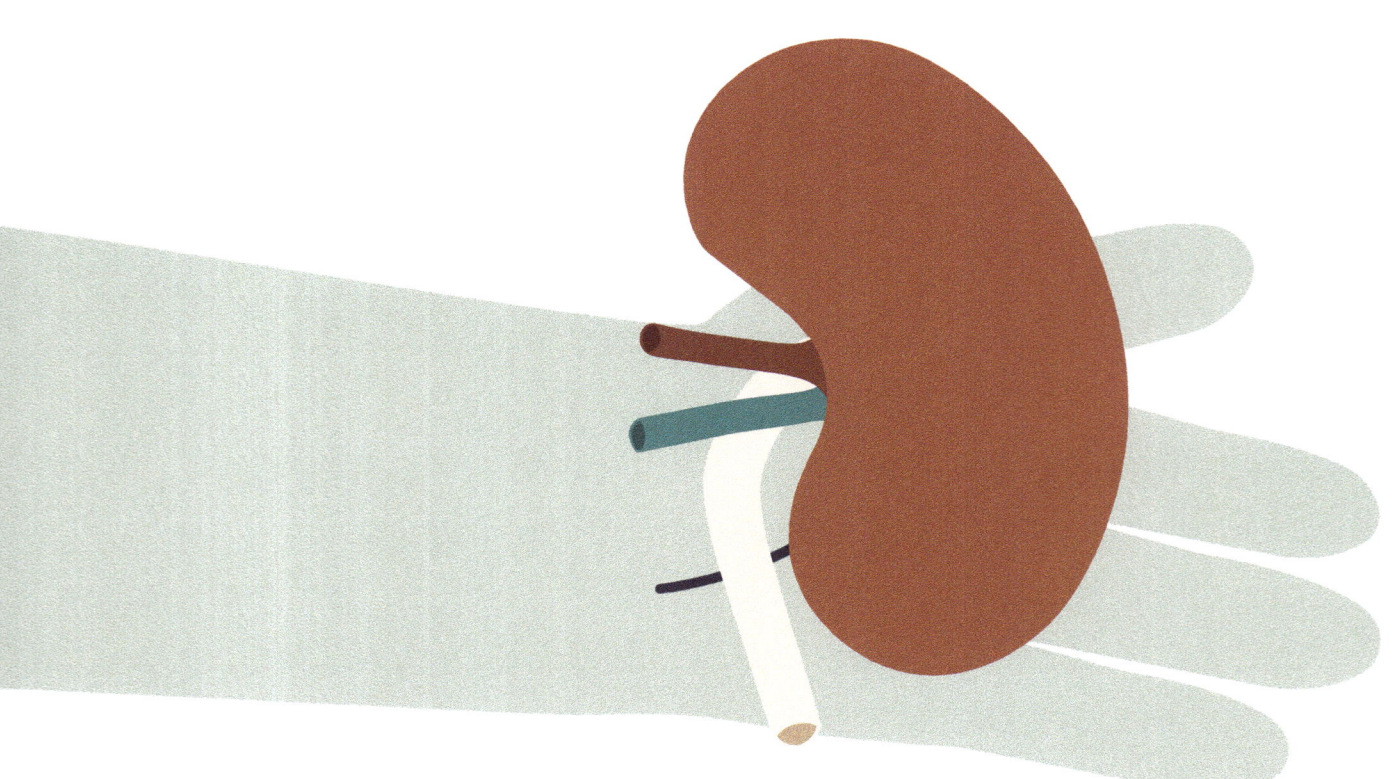

Or, a donor can be someone the person doesn't know.

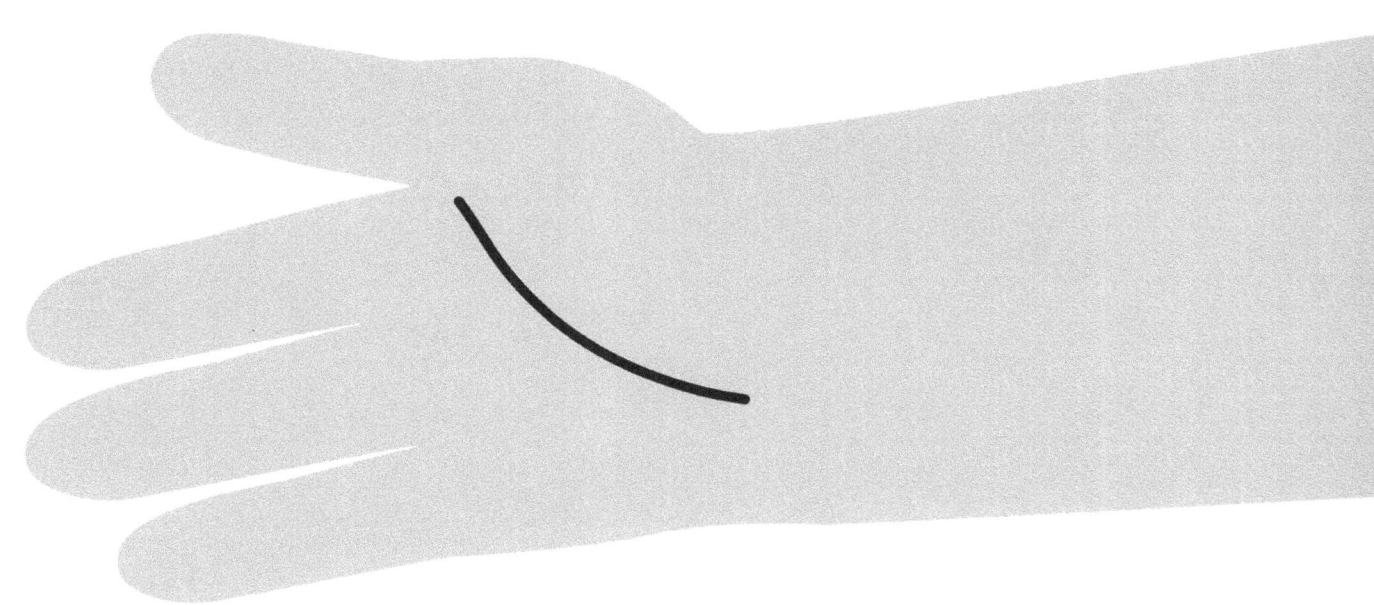

Do you know someone who needs a kidney?
Do you know where their kidney is coming from?

When the time comes for someone to get their new kidney, they will go to the hospital and have

surgery.

Surgery is when a doctor helps the inside of someone's body.

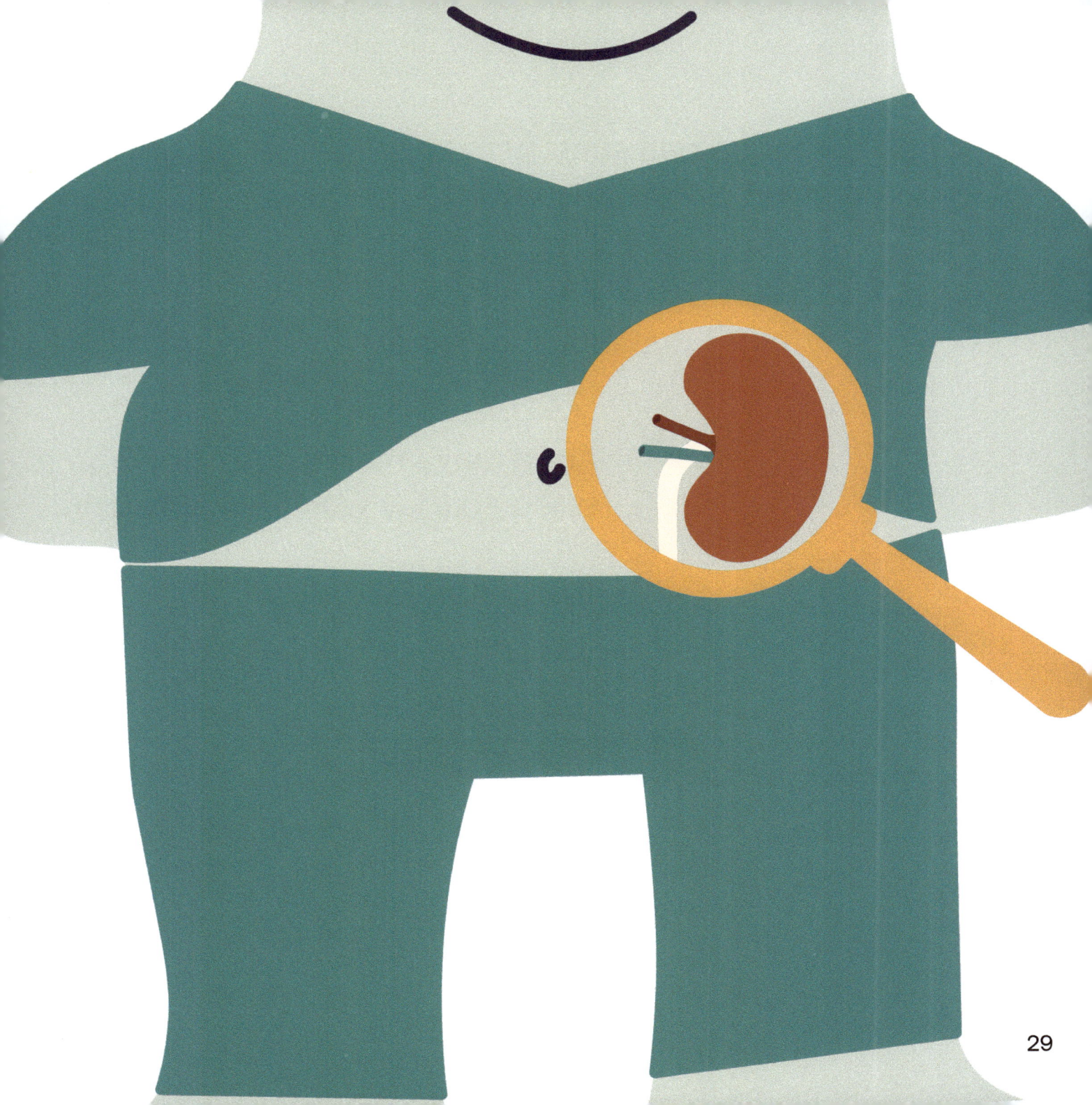

When someone has surgery,
they are given a medicine called

anesthesia

(sleepy medicine).

Anesthesia makes their body go to sleep so they won't feel anything.

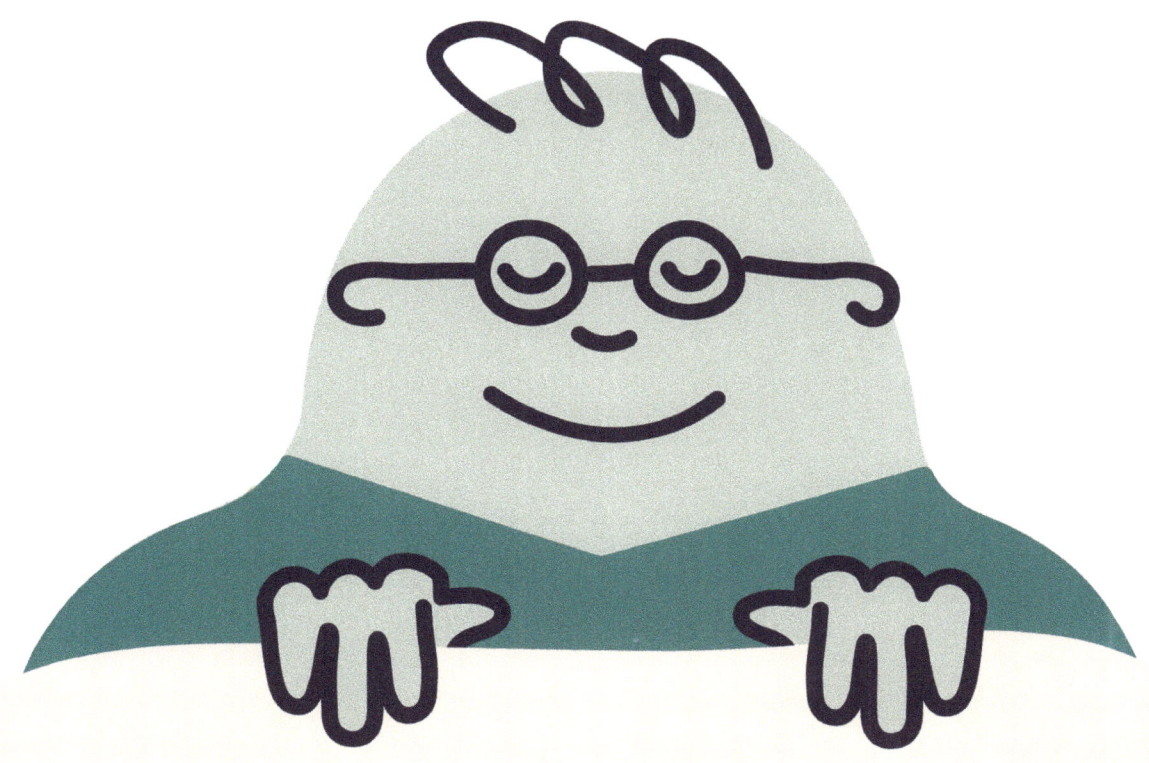

This kind of sleep is different than when someone goes to sleep on their own at night.

When the doctor stops giving the sleepy medicine their body wakes up.

During surgery, the doctor will disconnect the kidney that isn't working, and connect the new kidney.

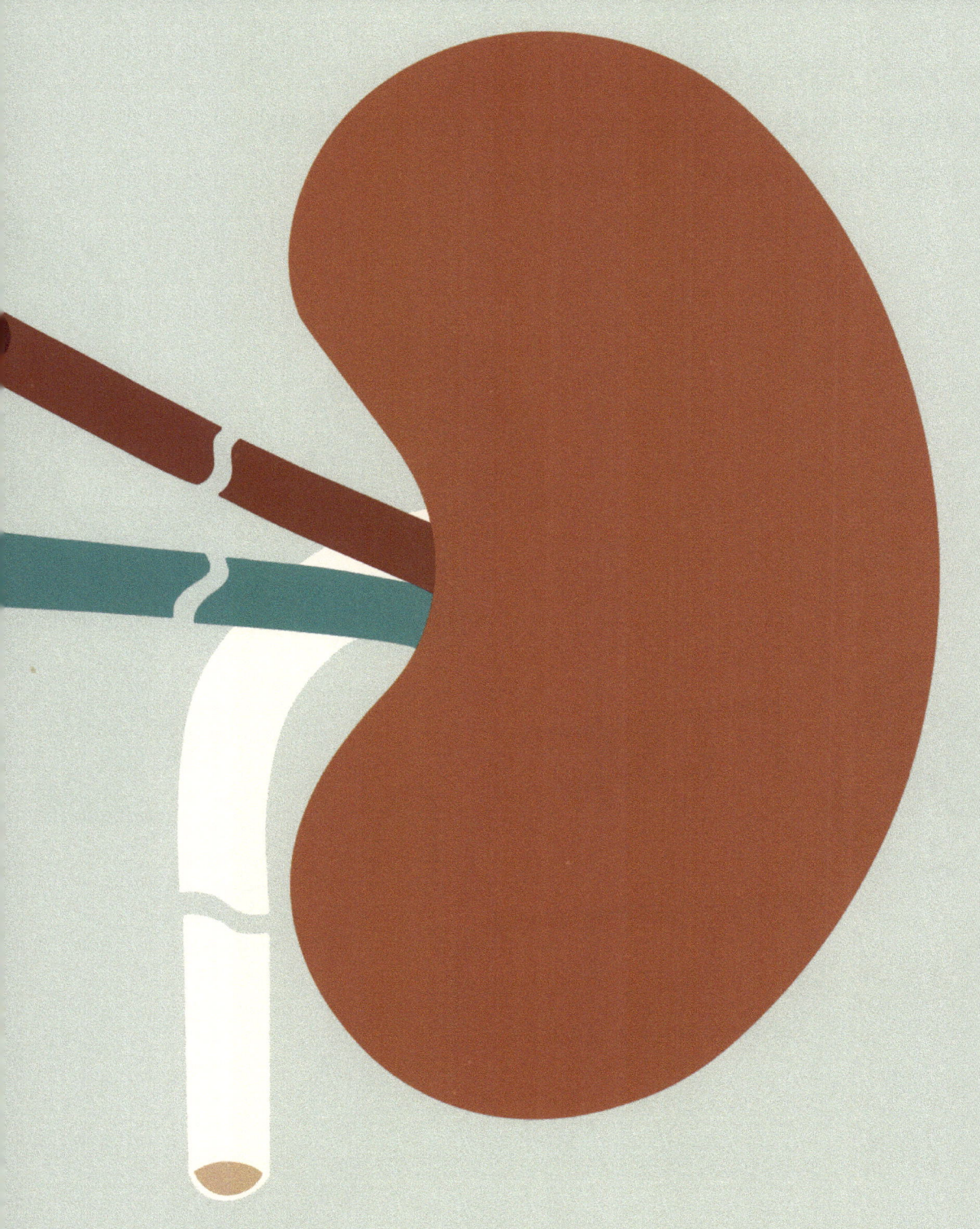

When someone gets a kidney transplant, they will have to rest their body in the hospital where they will be cared for by a team of people.

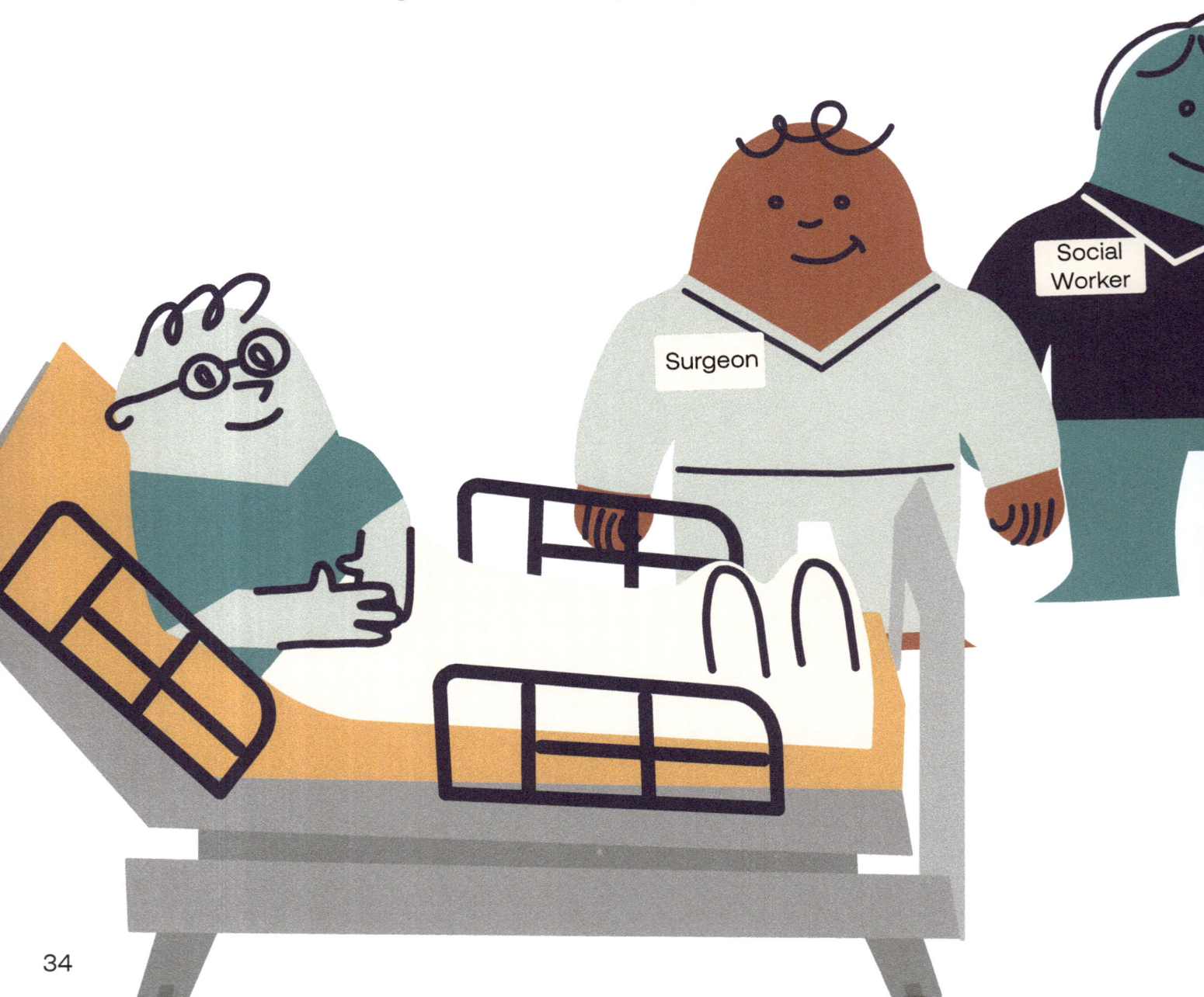

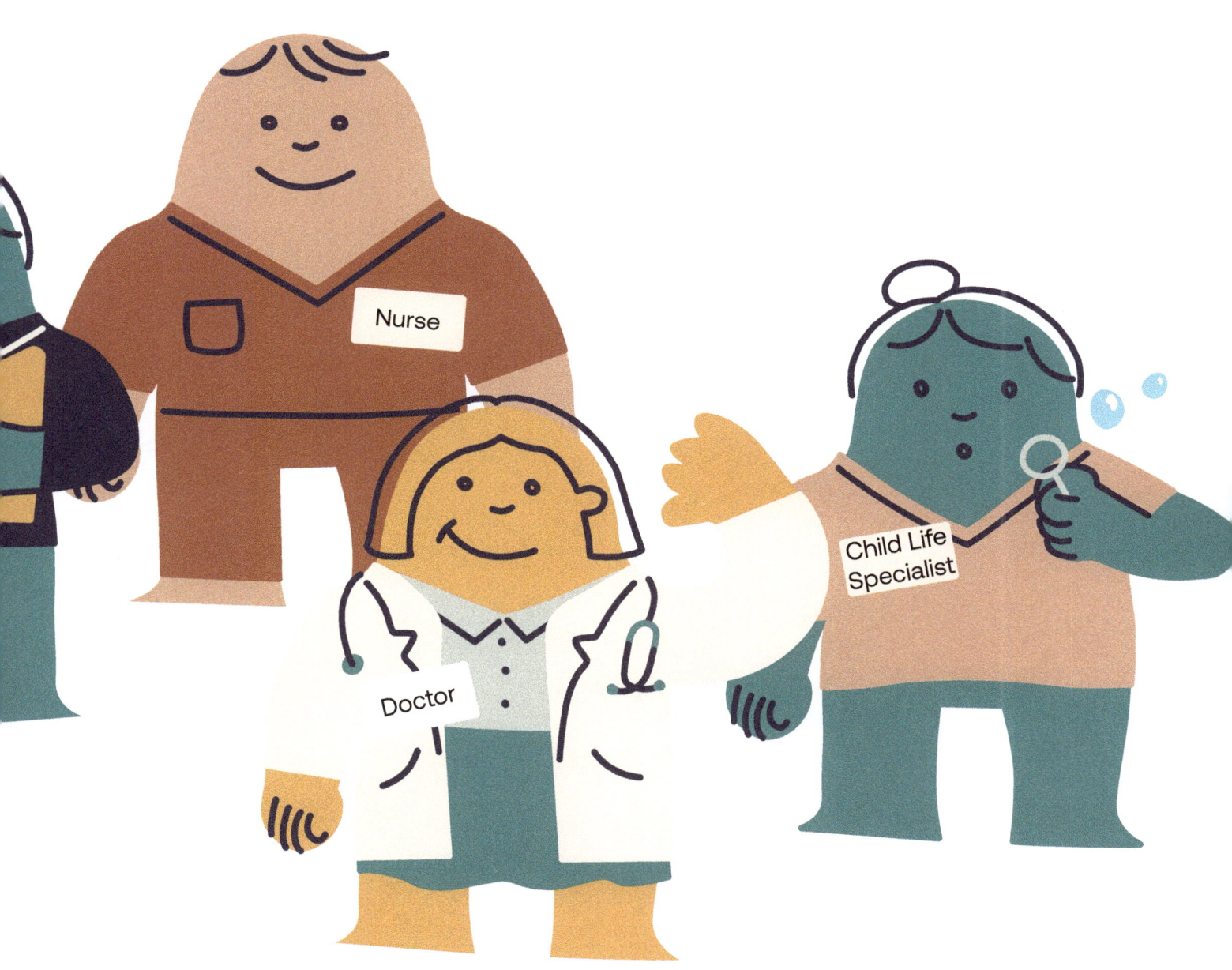

They will stay in the hospital until the doctors think they are ready to go home.

After someone gets a new kidney, they will have to do extra things to keep their new kidney healthy.

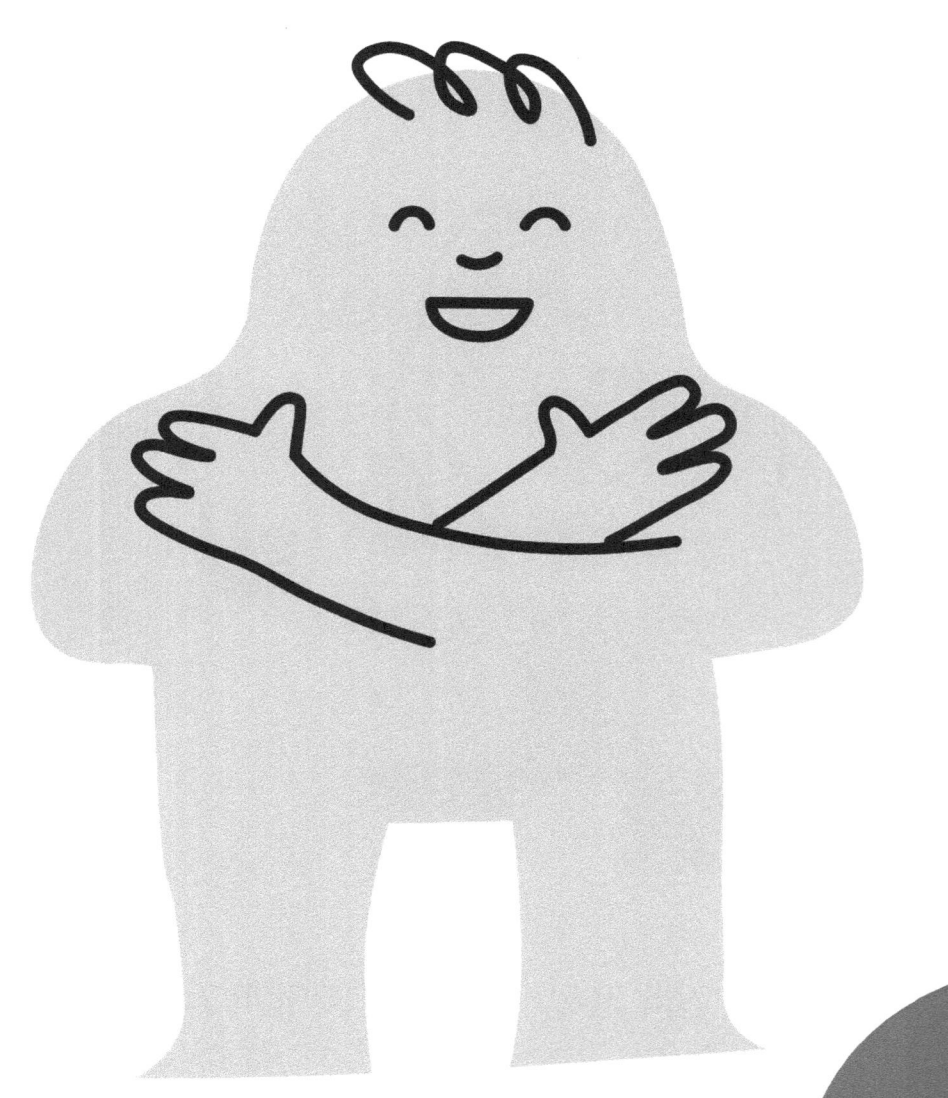

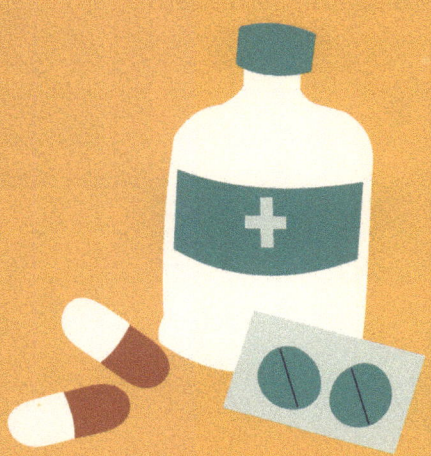

They will have to take medicine to keep the kidney strong,

and go visit the doctor to give the kidney a check-up.

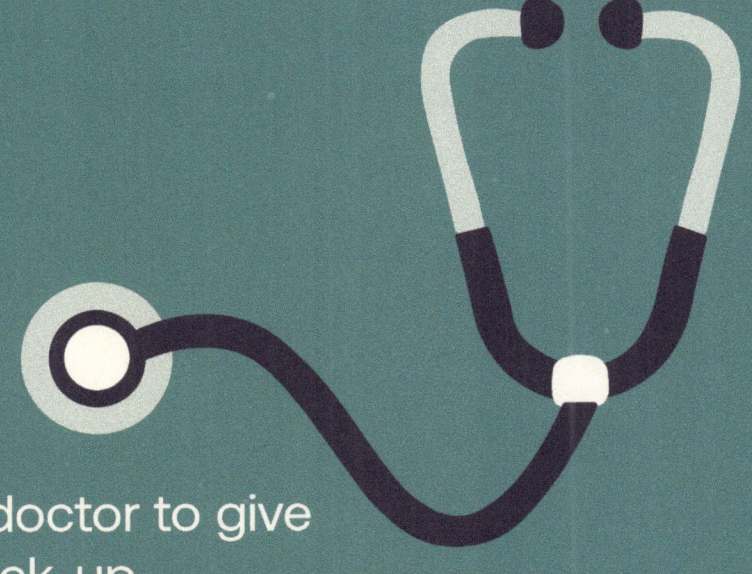

People with a kidney transplant can still do a lot of the things they enjoy doing, such as, eating their favorite food, riding their bike, or playing games with their friends.

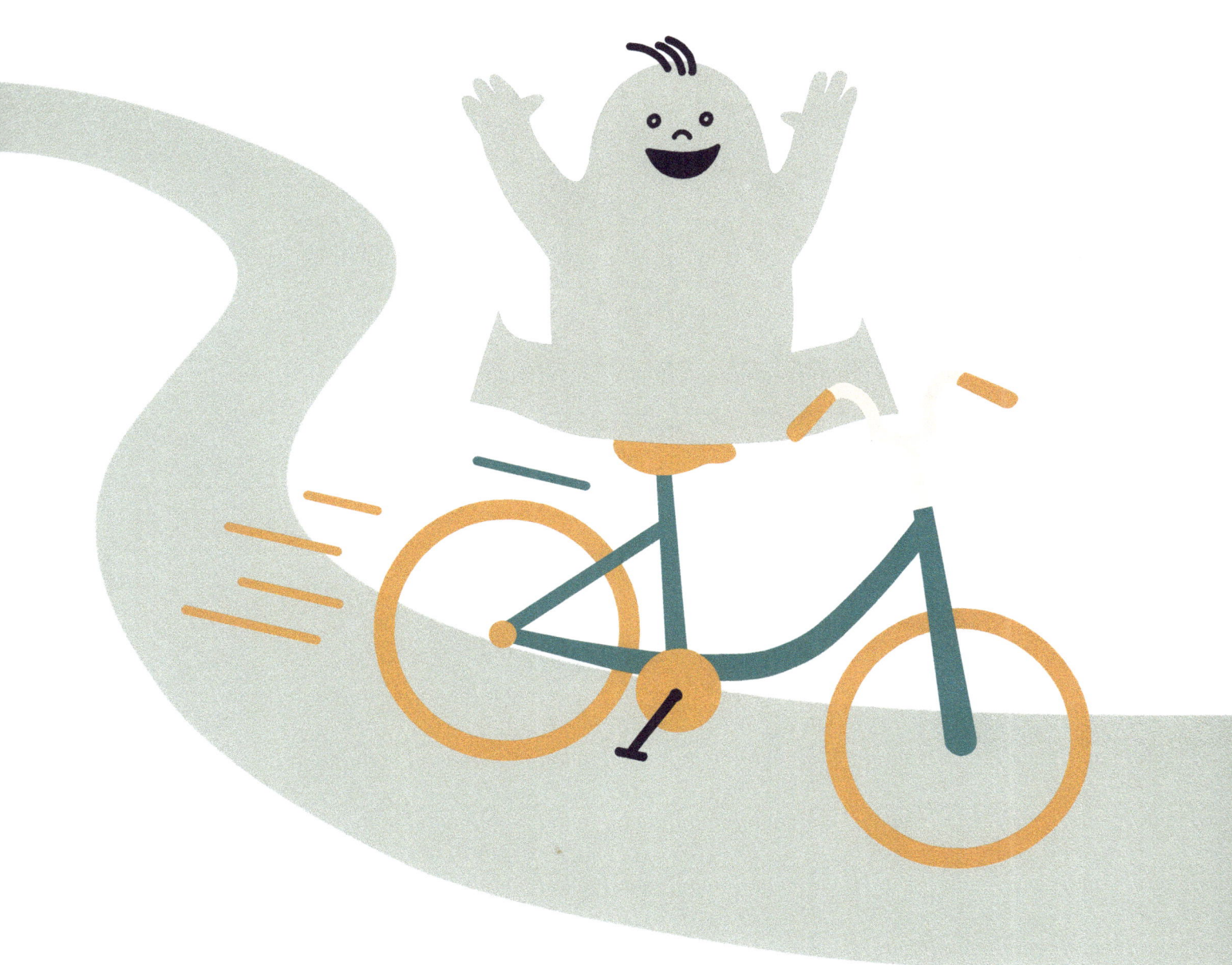

It can be helpful for someone with a new kidney to practice ahead of time what they want to share with their friends and family.

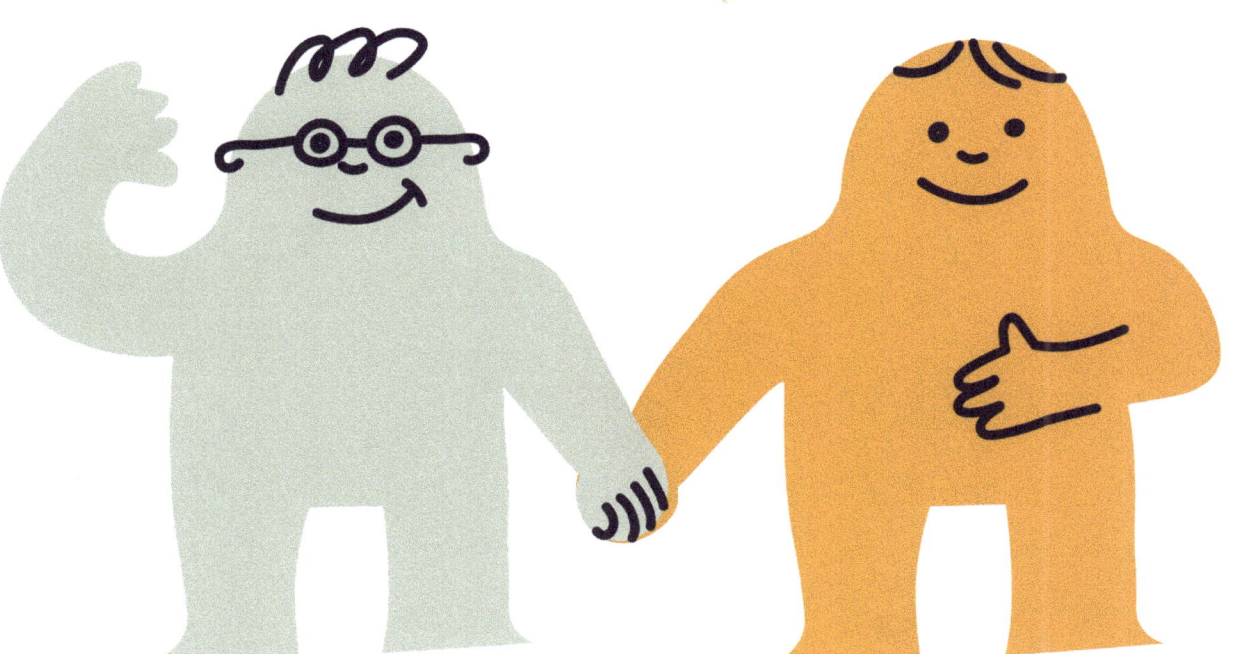

Wow, our bodies are pretty awesome!

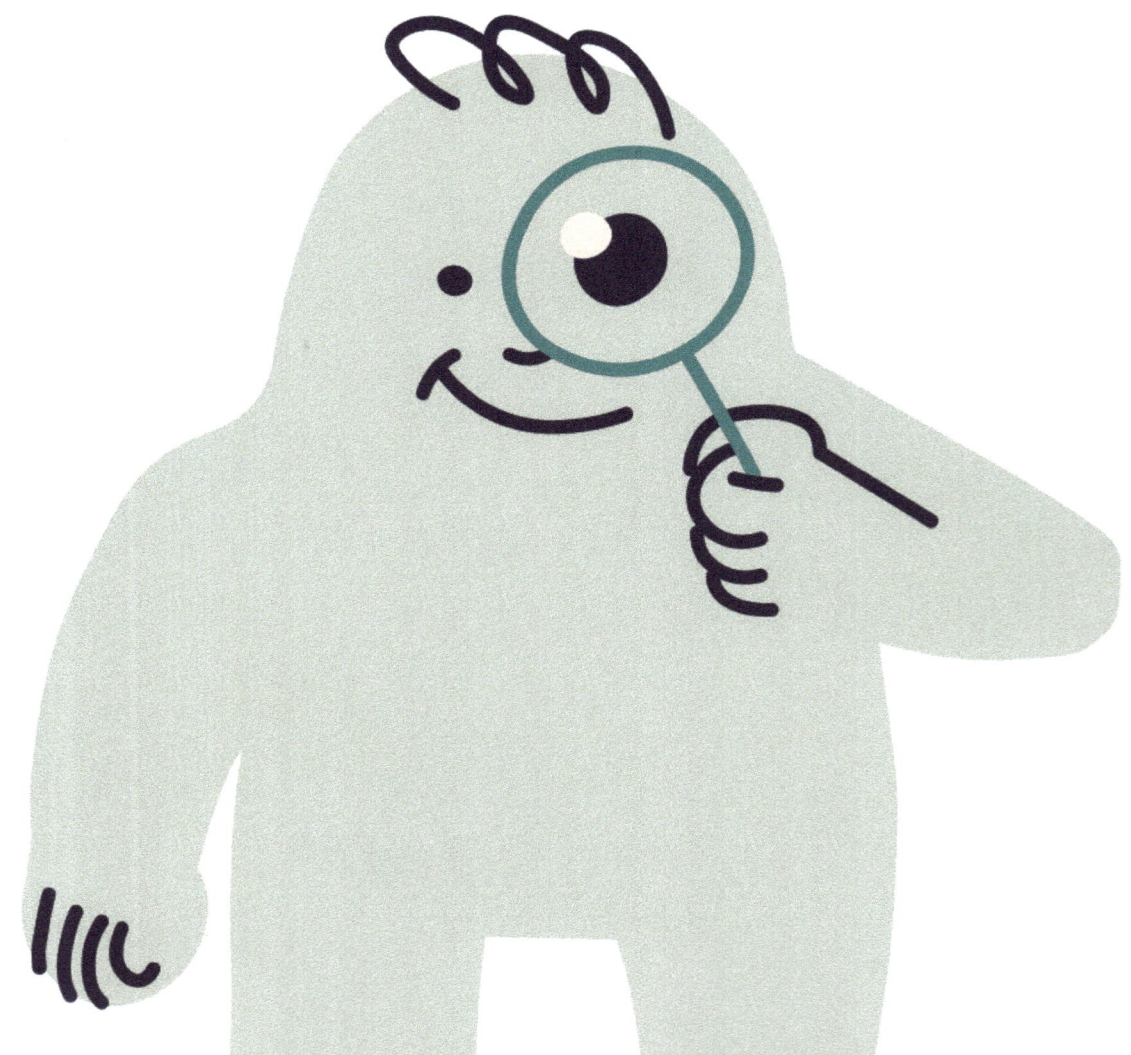

Now that we are experts in kidney transplants we can share what we have learned with our friends and family!

Glossary

Anesthesia

When someone has surgery, they are given a medicine called anesthesia. Anesthesia makes their body go to sleep so they won't feel, hear, or see anything. This kind of sleep is different than when someone goes to sleep on their own at night. When the doctor stops giving the sleepy medicine their body wakes up.

Donor

Organ donor: An organ donor is someone who donates, or gives, one of their body parts to someone else.

Living Organ Donor: A living organ donor is someone who chooses to give one of their organs to someone else when they are alive.

Deceased Organ Donor: A deceased organ donor is someone who wishes to give, or donate, their organs to someone else when they die. If someone chooses to be a deceased organ donor, the doctors can use any healthy organs that are not injured or impacted and give, or donate, them to someone who needs them.

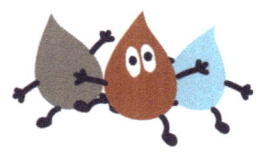

Fluid (of the body)

Our bodies need water (fluid) to stay healthy and make sure all of our organs and systems can do their jobs. Our kidneys use water to filter out waste from our blood. It then uses any extra fluid our body doesn't need to create urine (pee). Urine then carries the waste out of our body when we go to the bathroom.

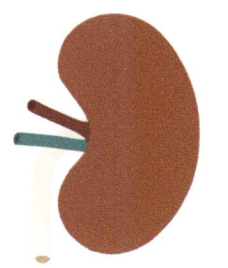

Kidney

Kidneys are bean shaped organs that are the size of our fist. They clean our blood and remove extra fluid and waste from our body. Then the extra fluid and waste leaves our body through our urine (pee). It is common for people to have two kidneys, but sometimes a body may only need one kidney to do the job of two.

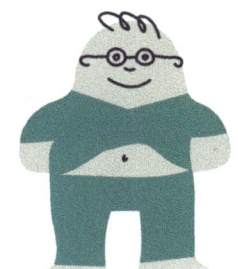

Surgery

Surgery is when a doctor helps the inside of someone's body.

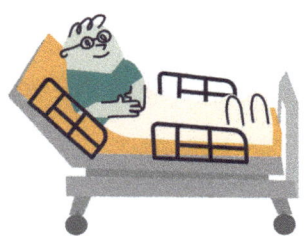

Transplant

Transplant means to move from one place to another, or relocate. When we are talking about our bodies, transplant means moving one organ, or body part, from one person to another. This can help to replace a damaged or sick body part with a new, healthy body part.

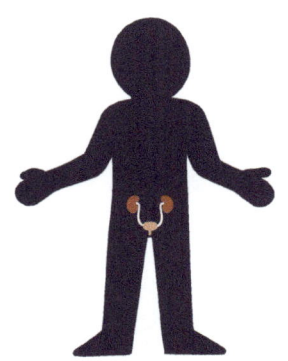

Urinary System

The urinary system is the group of body parts (organs) that all work together to clean the body's blood and make urine. It is common for the urinary system to be made up of two kidneys, two ureters, one bladder and one urethra, but sometimes, a urinary system may only have one kidney.

Waste (of the body)

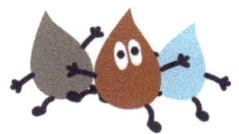

Things that collect in our bodies that we don't need to keep us healthy. They can include pieces of broken down food that our bodies don't need, cells that don't work anymore, parts of germs that have been defeated, and/or extra vitamins.

Do you know someone who needs to take extra care of their kidneys?

(here is where you can talk about someone you know who has a kidney related diagnosis, or is in the process of a kidney transplant)

Can you think of activities that children can do while waiting in a hospital or at a doctor's visit?

(draw or make a list of activities you think of here)

Kidney Maze!

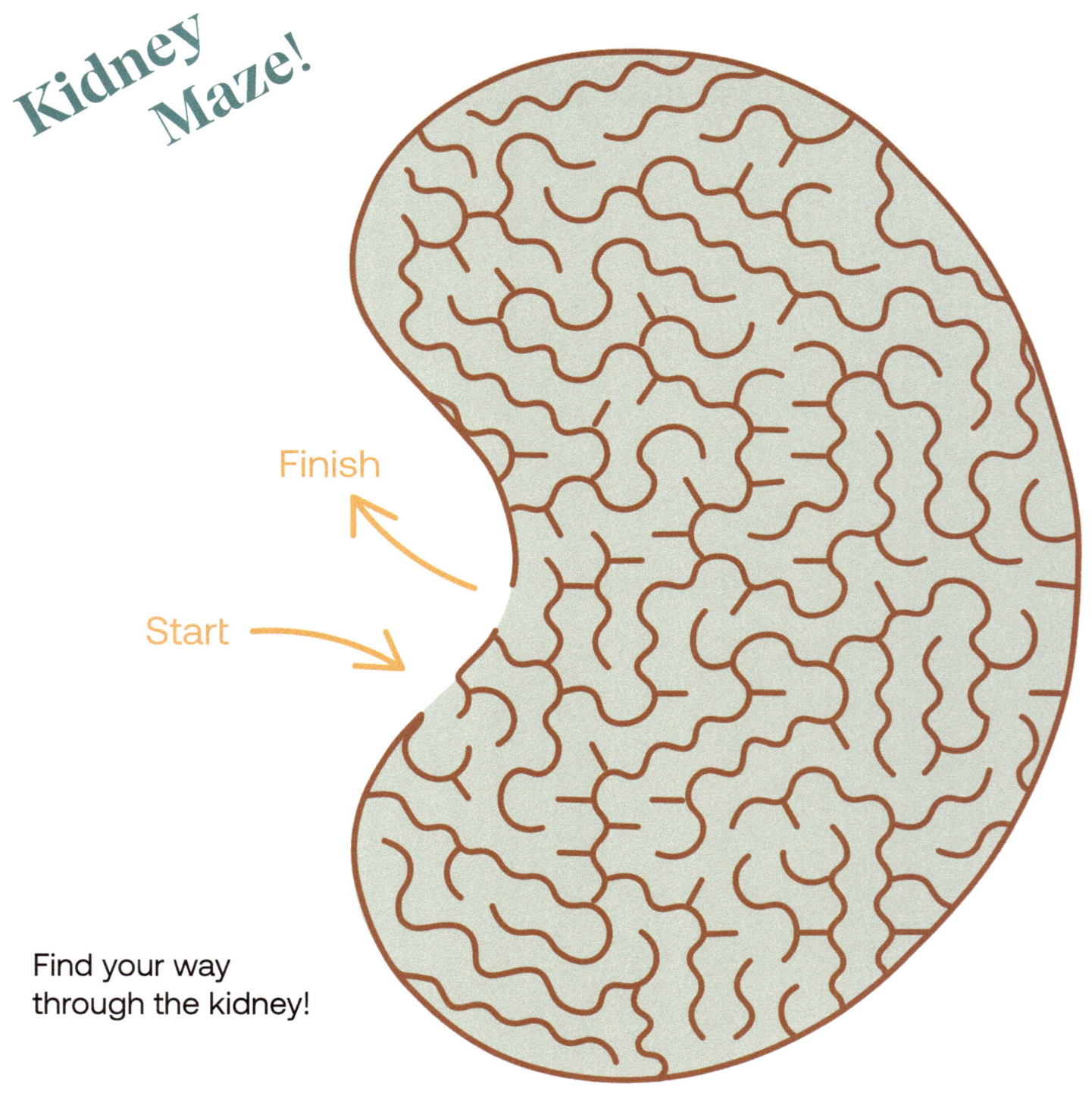

Find your way through the kidney!

Kidney Filtration Activity:

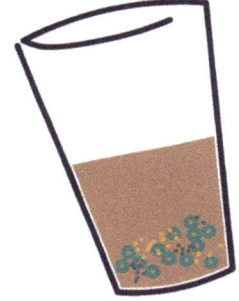
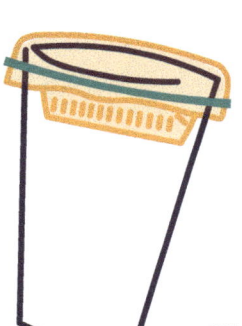

It is helpful for children to be introduced to new topics, especially abstract topics like the job of the kidney, through hands-on activities. This can include, books, art projects, and/or through play.

The Kidney Filtration Activity is a great activity to do in partnership with this book. It can aid in children's learning and understanding of how the kidneys do their job of filtering fluid and waste out of the blood.

This activity can be done for general learning purposes, for children needing a kidney transplant, and/or for children who know someone who needs a new kidney.

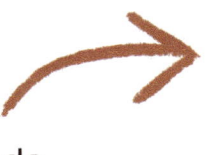

For printable instructions:
Use your phone's camera to scan the QR code,
or visit www.childcorefamilysupport.com/kidney-filtration-activity/

About the Authors

Child Core Family Support is a Child Life Specialist run company that provides consultation, resources, and information to caregivers of children going through medical experiences as well as support for providers who serve these families.

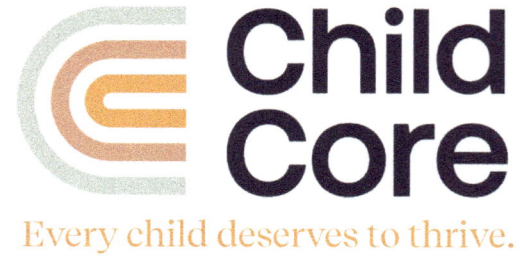

Their educational library strives to equip caregivers and professionals with the tools to feel confident and empowered when supporting a child through medical complexities. Child Core also offers free caregiver guides for talking to a child about a medical experience, and 1:1 coaching to meet the unique needs of individual families.

Find more information, resources, or to learn about child life specialists visit our WEBSITE.